The Single Man's Guide to Self Satisfaction

Dr Richard O'Nan and Pamela Palm

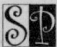

SP

SUMMERSDALE

First published 1997.

ISBN 1 84024 109 8

Summersdale Publishers Ltd
46 West Street
Chichester
West Sussex
PO19 1RP

www.summersdale.com

Printed and bound in Great Britain

Contents

God created the male orgasm so Adam would know when to stop

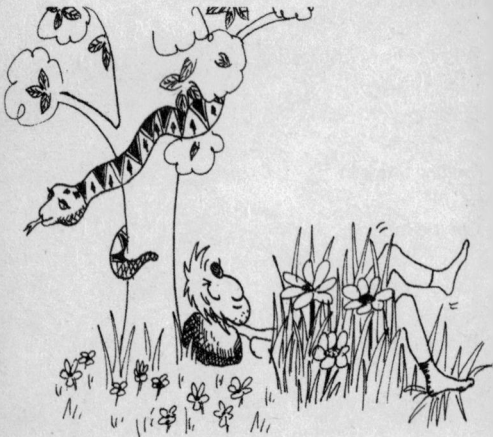

Introduction

Girlfriend just left you? Can't [be bothered to] get a girlfriend? Or maybe you've just got a few minutes to spare: time on your hands, so to speak? Whatever the situation, men - this book is for you.

Men want sex; women want romance, attention, children, money, someone to stand around while they try on clothes they don't like, arguments and a great divorce settlement. An oversimplification? Perhaps. Sure, men want other stuff too - heck, we've all got a sensitive side. But what if sex with yourself could be just as much fun as sex with another person or people? You could have great sex whenever you wanted, as often as you wanted, and without having to sit up and beg for it. Interested? Then read on . . .

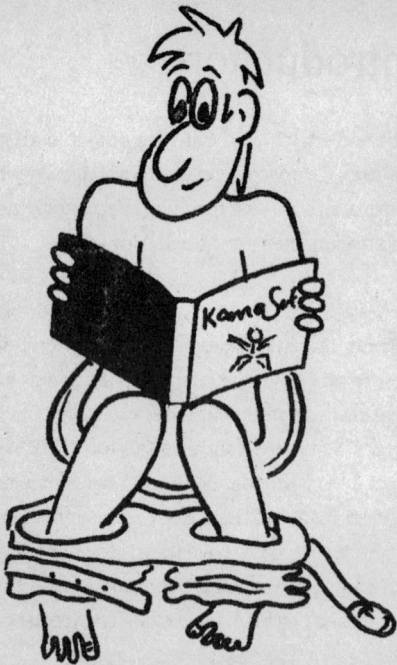

A Brief History of Tossing . . .

Ever since the first caveman stopped bashing his wife over the head and started beating his meat instead, progress and the penis have gone hand in hand. Sex-crazed simians bent on working up a better head of steam than four paws and a prehensile tail could achieve - these are the heroes of our race.

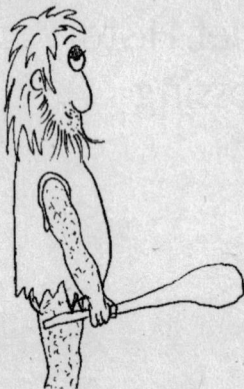

Why the dinosaurs became extinct

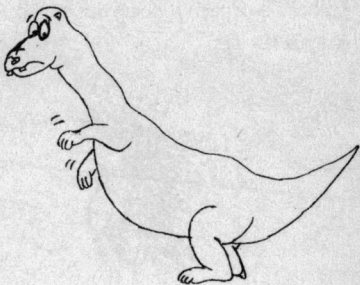

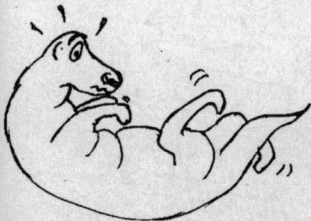

The only exception was the invention of fire - the direct result of the Neantherthal masturbatory technique of palm rubbing being tried with sticks by jealous females.

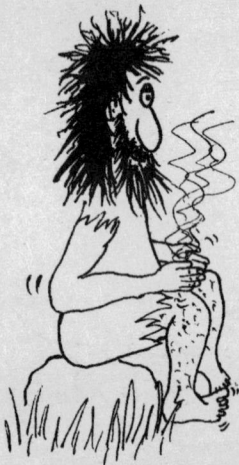

What indeed was the spur to human evolution if not the opposable thumb?

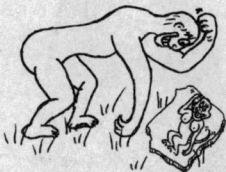

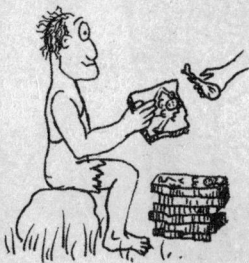

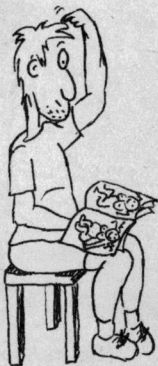

The past has much to teach the persistent palmist . .

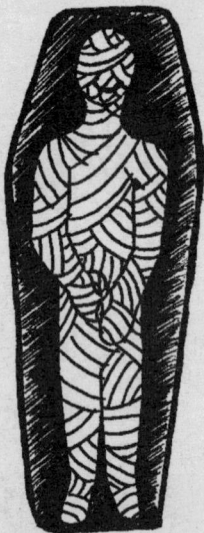

The happy afterlife - Egyptian style

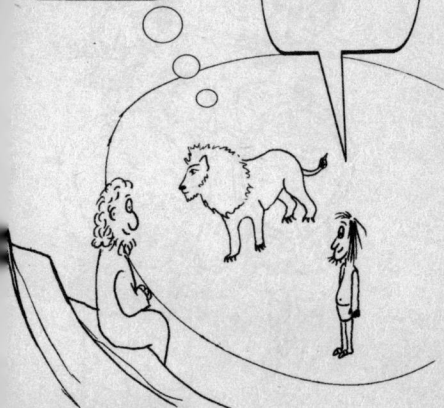

The Vikings were proud of their helmets

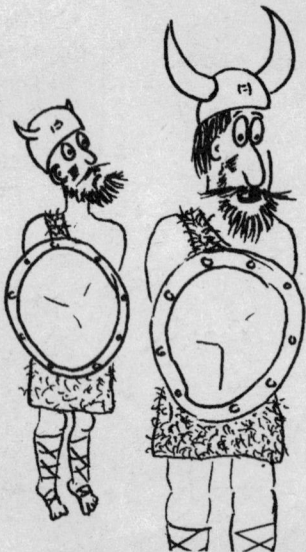

The Armoured Codpiece

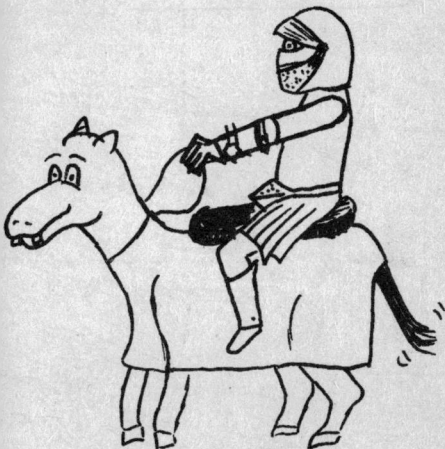

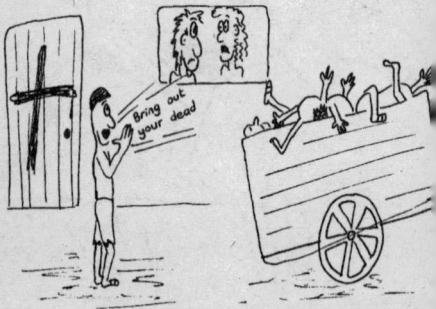

The Discovery of America

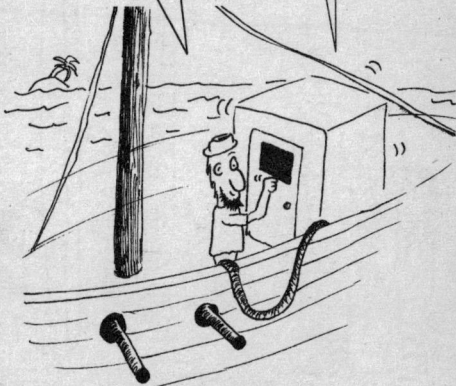

The French Revolution

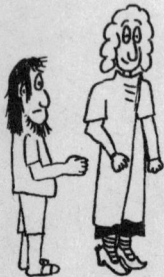

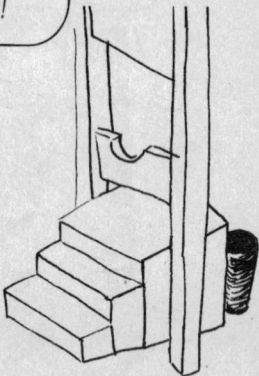

Custer's Last Stand

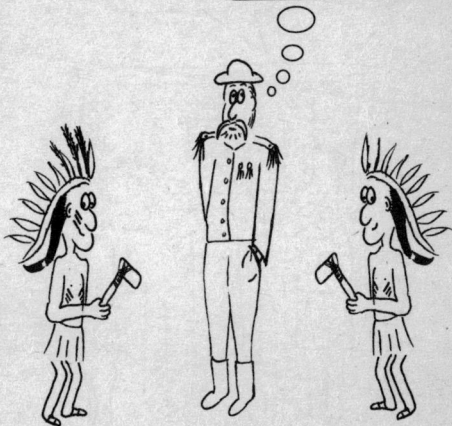

The Great British Empire

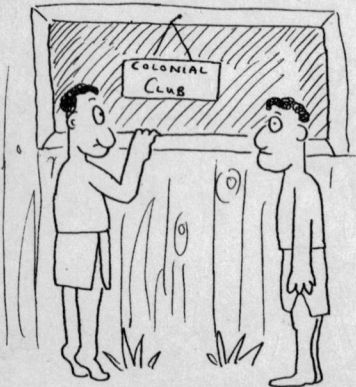

Any history of men pleasing themselves has to pay homage, of course, to the great Victorian inventor, cheesemaker and master masturbator, John Thomas Entwhistle, who devoted his life to developing the ultimate tossing machine.

Entwhistle's Self-Manipulating Frottalogicon, as he called it, was an ingenious creation that, through a well-oiled system of gears, fan-belts and rubber wheels, converted the brisk turning of a simple hand crank into a violent pistoning effect of over one hundred pumps per second. By manipulating a series of foot pedals, the intrepid operator increased or decreased frottalogic intensity and barometric pressure, while saucy picture postcards were displayed in sequence through a viewing tube.

After Entwhistle's untimely and excessively violent death 'at the wheel', Henry Ford succeeded in developing a mobile version of the Frottalogicon that has kept wankers on the road ever since.

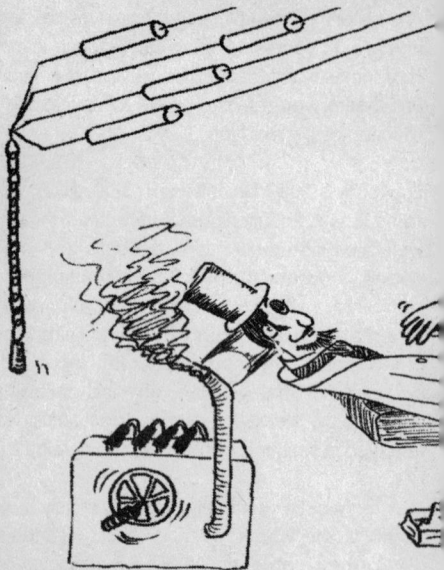

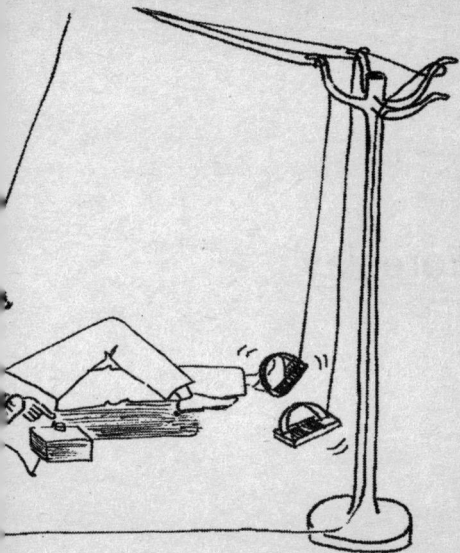

An Early Prototype of the Frottalogicon

Foreplay

When young couples laugh and skip through the trees and meadows, their eyes full only of love for each other, society calls this romance. But if a single man, full of love for himself, were to do the same, society would come down on him like a ton of bricks, several hundreds of tons, in fact, in the form of an institution for the incontinentally insane. As a result, men have locked away their natural romantic feelings of self-love, and many, I fear to say, even abuse themselves.

But there can be romance, indeed, there must be romance in a self-sexual relationship if you are ever to get really in touch with yourself.

So repeat after me the following mantra for male masturbators everywhere:

> I think a lot of myself.
> I think I'm so special.
> I really fancy myself something rotten.

Feels good, huh?

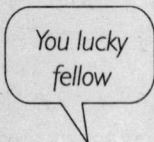

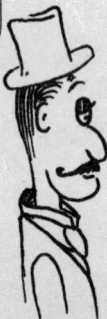

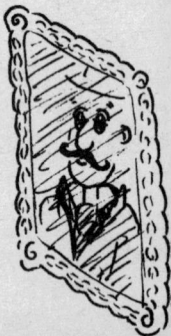

You lucky fellow

Take yourself out for a meal:

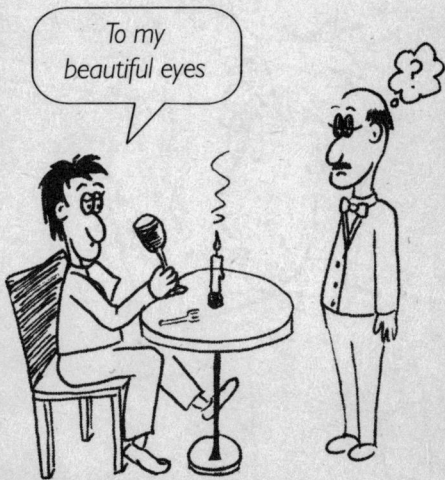

Why not try chatting yourself up in a pub or a club?

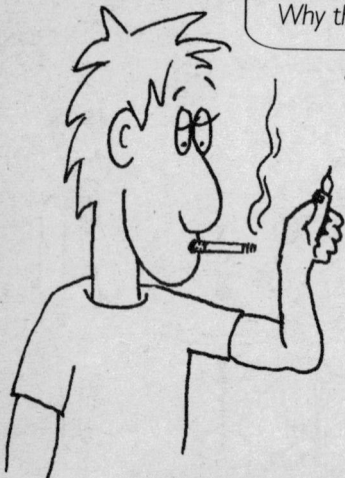

Or just buy yourself a present after a hard day's work:

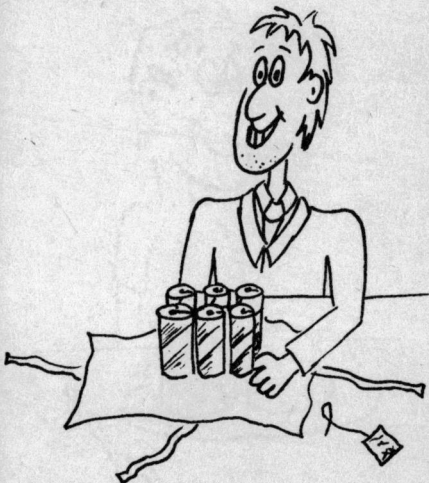

For the dedicated pleasure seeker, aphrodisiac meals for one can be a real turn on:

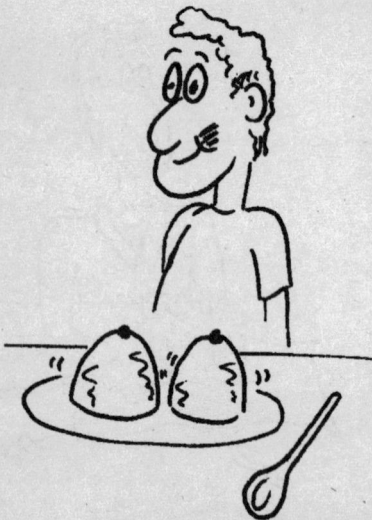

Warming Up

All athletes will tell you the importance of warming up if you are to achieve your peak speed and flexibility - and avoid injuries that could really put a dampner on your quality time. Experts from the University of Essex have developed some excellent exercises that warm up your wrist, forearm and elbow, and improve flexibility and stamina more generally.

Exercise One: Cup both hands, palms facing upwards, and flex all fingers and both thumbs inwards and outwards, as though checking a couple of melons for ripeness.

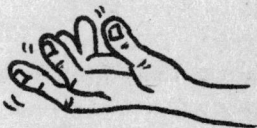

Exercise Two: Curl your fingers round and touch your thumb to your first finger. Move your hand rapidly back and forwards from the wrist and elbow, trying to achieve the most fluid movement. This valuable exercise can be performed anywhere: many people seem to enjoy using it even in moving traffic.

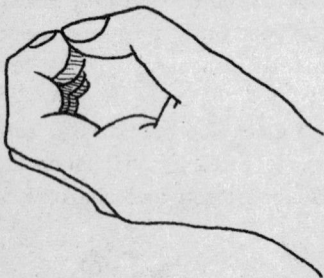

Exercise Three: Take a phone directory and roll it up as tightly as you can. This exercise builds stamina essential for the long haul.

Perfect Penile Potential

The world's greatest tossers seek to achieve PPP - Perfect Penile Potential. By combining a carefully-chosen diet with rigorous exercise, careful massage and a plentiful supply of Scandinavian erotica, these heroes of the art can keep themselves on the boil continually for the ninety hour marathon that marks the climax of the Wankalympics. While few can aspire to such feats, there are several techniques we can usefully learn from such marvels of modern manhood.

1) A **daily massage** with aromatherapy massage oils will keep your old man in top working condition, and helps guard against friction burns - which nobody wants.

2) **Sports psychology** - it is very important to stay in contact with your penis throughout the working day. Most men achieve this publicly, though often subconsciously, by continuously petting and fondling themselves through their trouser pockets, by frequent hoisting up of their trousers, and by scratching their bollocks. In these troubled times, wopping it out whenever you feel the urge is not, sadly, to be recommended.

3) **Mental agility** - the greatest tossers are those whose brains have become totally fixated by sex. As boys, we all saw the world entirely through sex-tinted glasses - we must seek to recapture this golden age.

You must strive to find sexual connotations in the most innocent of phrases. Try saying the following: 'I can't seem to open this door: the knob's a bit stiff.' Did you smirk with schoolboy glee at the naughty double meaning? Well done! But you still have some way to go. Champion wankers can go on for hours just at the thought of two milk bottles and a packet of scampi fries.

4) **Yoga** - study the following positions from the secret teachings of Jacques Oeuf, the famous French self-sexualist.

The Weathervane

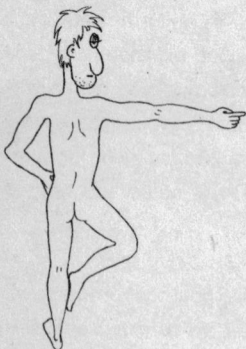

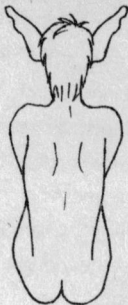

The Roaring Bull

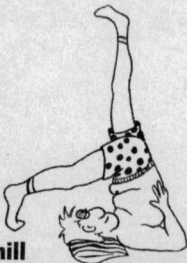

The Windmill

Getting Stuck In

Every home provides a great deal of scope for sexual experimentation by the single man, so kick the cat out, lock the doors, close the curtains, and get stuck in . . .

Artificial Stimulation

There are artificial aids available to enhance your lovelife: best known of which is the blow-up doll, the sex mate who is always willing and ready. Although your mates will laugh if they find your latex love interest tucked behind the sofa, they will be secretly envious of your trouble-free sex life - no arguments about what to watch on TV, no foreplay, and no way you can fail to satisfy!

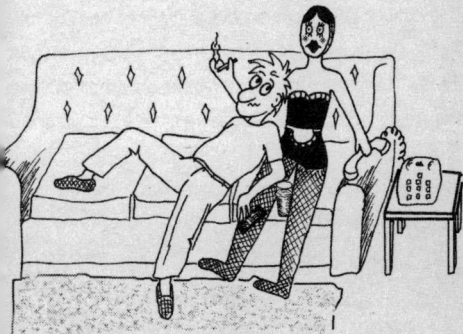

Bliss in inflatable form though it may be, you can get a lot more out of your blow-up doll than sex alone. You can have a fulfilling relationship - with the only pressure being her pounds per square inch. Some sexy lingerie from Oxfam, a meal for two (keep the candles over your side of the table).

Gaze into her eyes, seduce her. Don't take her silence as rejection: it is desire so deep it strikes her dumb.

Kiss her long and hard, undress each other slowly (she might need some help here).

Result - adoration. And if she demands commitment, you can just pull the plug.

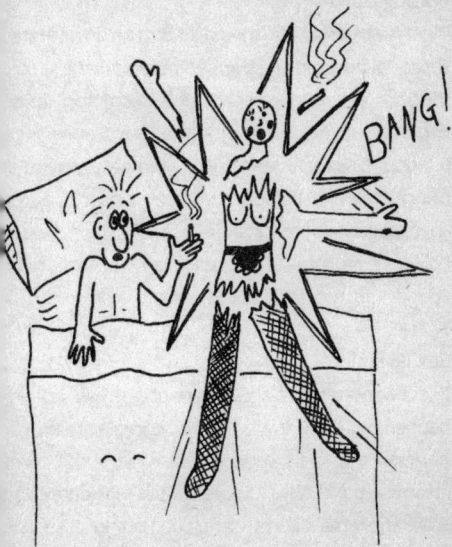

BANG!

Pornography

Most men would give their right arm for an unlimited supply of good strong porn. Where, indeed, would modern society be without it? But it can be so expensive. The videos, internet hard core sites, telephone sex lines and imported magazines are as out of reach for the less well-heeled onanist as top shelf magazines are for short arses. There are ways, however, to simulate your own red hot Amsterdam shopping spree, for a fraction of the cost.

Sex lines

If you want to spend ages on the phone with nothing happening, then any customer complaint line can perform the same service. But what about some steamy action?! Any plumber will talk for hours about male and female parts, or ring up your local kennels about bitches on heat, or inquire at the cattery about your next door neighbour's pussy.

Sex scenes

For your own home-made hardcore porn film, buy a notepad, then draw a slightly different pose on each bottom right corner: a rapid ruffle through the pages, and there you have it - non-stop red hot porno, flick book style! For the less artistic, simply stick nude bodies cut from jazz mags or fine art catalogues onto your television screen; line them up with the head of the newsreader of your choice, and let your imagination go.

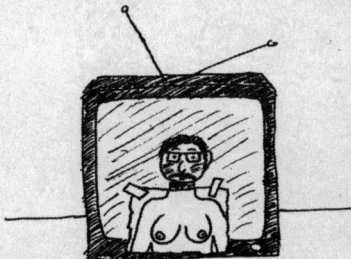

Peep Shows

Go to an art exhibition wearing a cardboard box over your head (don't worry, you will not look out of place). Find a nude statue or painting of frolicking nymphs, and observe the anatomy bit by bit through your eyehole.

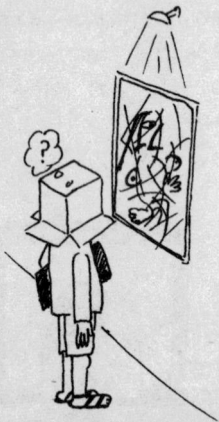

›sitions

ecent surveys of solitary sexual behaviour have
own that the Western male uses a rather limited
nge of positions when engaged in solo sex.
ompare this with the two thousand, four hundred
d nineteen basic positions outlined in the classic
dian text on self-satisfaction, the Sadd Oo 'Anka. In
e time it takes an 'Anka initiate to complete the
st three stages of awakening (up to eyebrow
mulation), the average Western man is already
wn the pub and on his second pint.

hile there is nothing wrong with the old favourites,
ere are many variations to be experimented with
r those spicier evenings alone.

rn your own home into a harem . . .

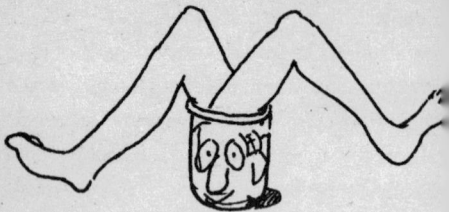

Eastern techniques

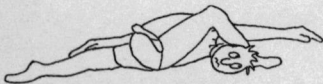

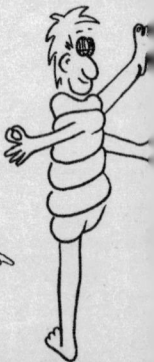

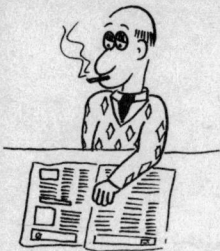

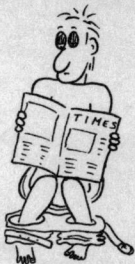

Western techniques

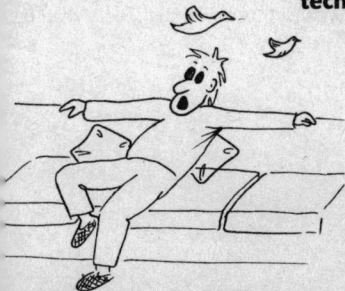

The range of stimulating locations within the humble home is simply mindblowing! And the great thing about the single man's sex life is that it can be combined with all those jobs that every man hates to do . . .

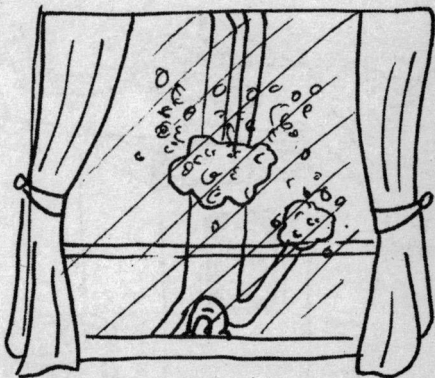

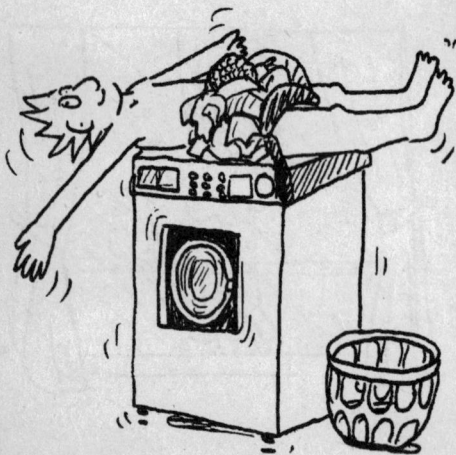

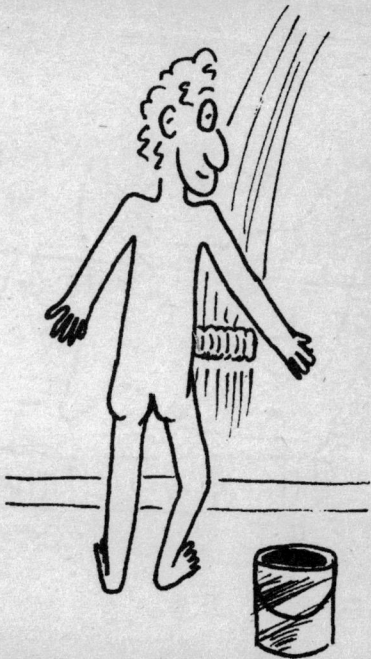

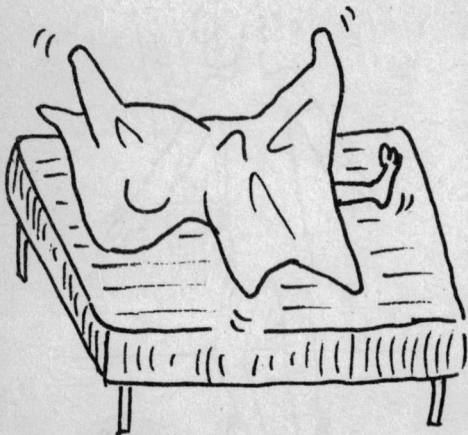

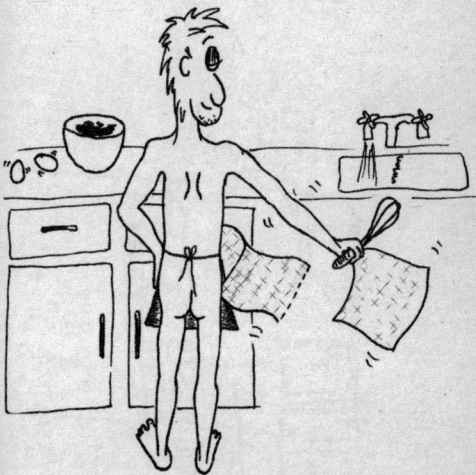

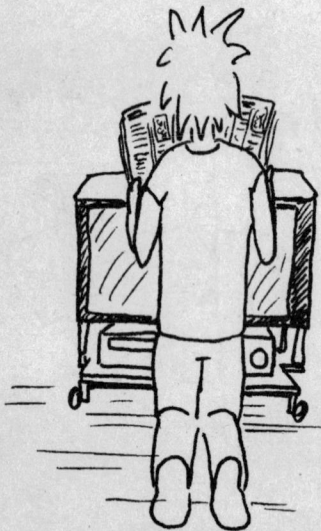

bleep!
bleep!

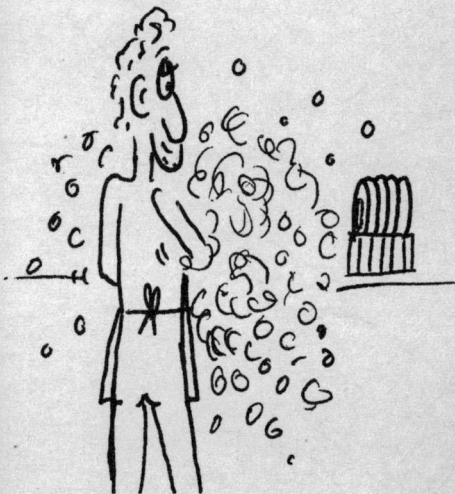

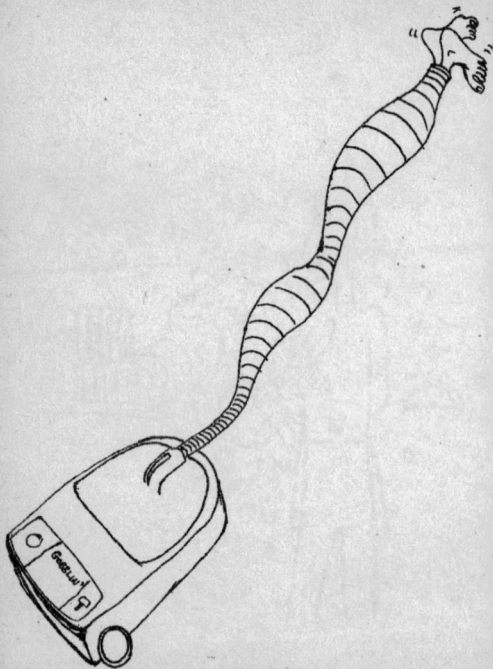

On the Job

As anyone will tell you, there are always wankers wherever you work. There is a very good psychological reason for this: at work, men can express the personalities they wished they had - overconfident, arrogant, all-knowing sporting heroes with a sex life that Hollywood stars would envy. This is true for married, attached and single men alike - until the wife or girlfriend turns up. Then it is a very different story. Only the single man can hold onto his dreams: women have the habit of turning them into delusions.

At the office, a man's dreams can remain intact. Where better, then, to expand your sexual relationship with yourself? If you can be a different person at work, then that means that, as a single man, you can have sex with your different self. Good, eh?

Due to the small-mindedness of the legal system, it is inadvisable to display your self-satisfying skills before your work colleagues. Discretion is paramount, and you should always be aware of the potentially life-changing consequences of your work-time activities coming into the open.

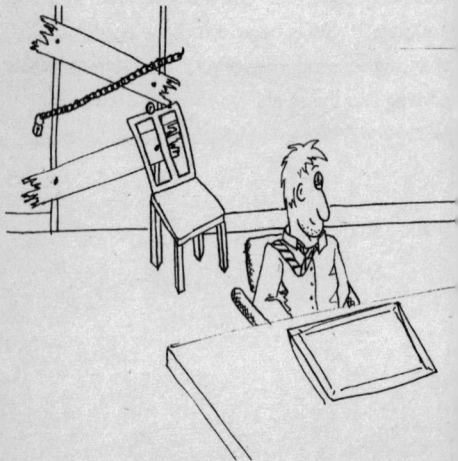

Many office managers get over this problem by having weights or cycling machines in a corner of their office as a way of explaining why they are so often red in the face and panting slightly when you knock on their door. For those lower down the corporate ladder, you can always try the 'it's an exercise to combat the effects of repetitive stress syndrome' line, or, if things are rather more advanced, say you spilt the Tippex.

The Health and Safety Officer

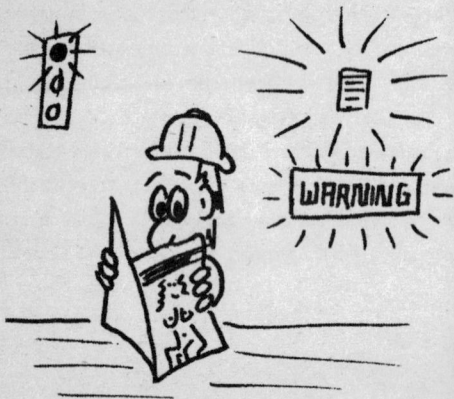

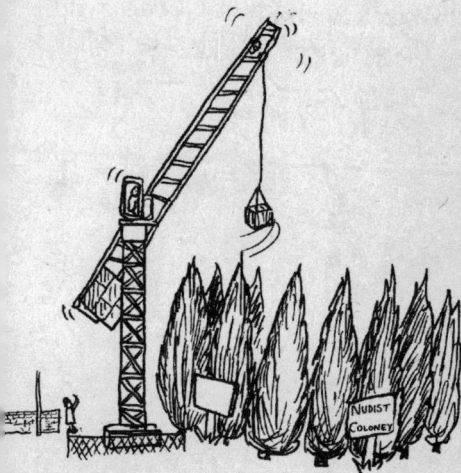

NUDIST COLONEY

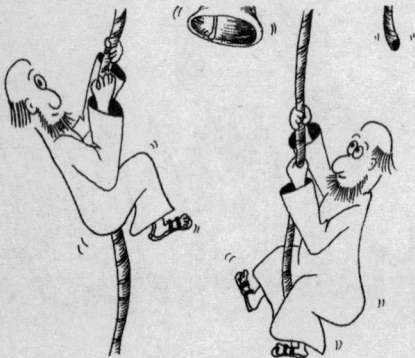

The Car Jack

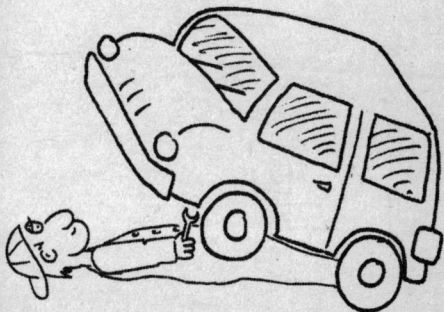

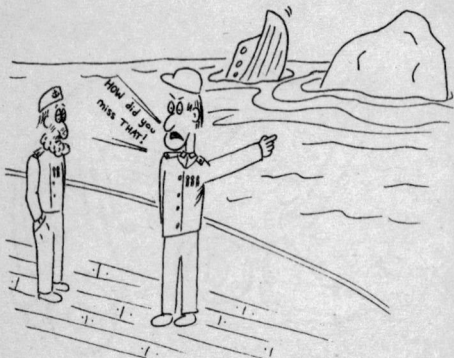

The Checkout

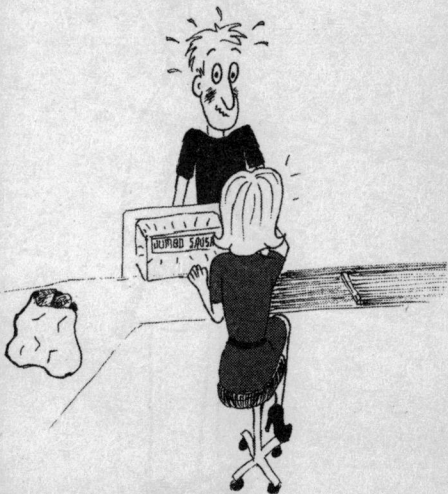

Bobby on the beat

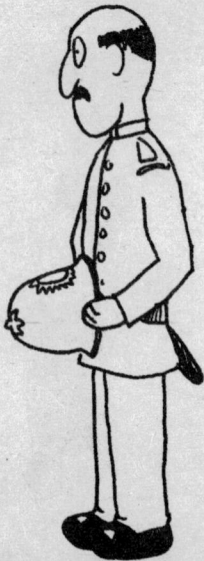

Pizza base tosser

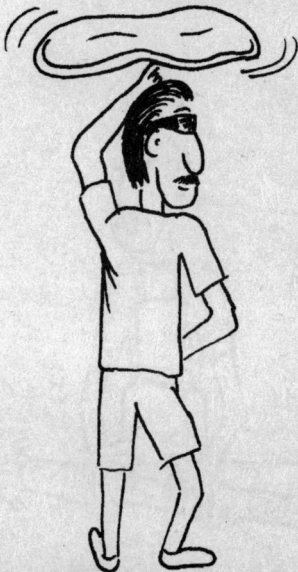

Kneading the French Stick

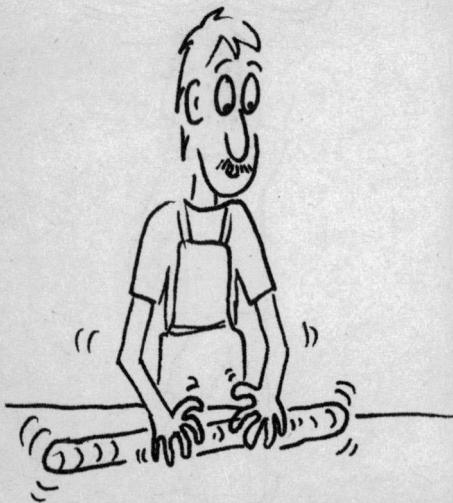

Pilot Error

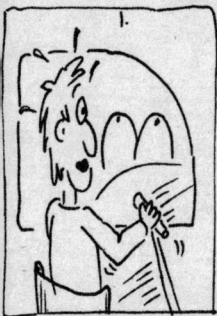

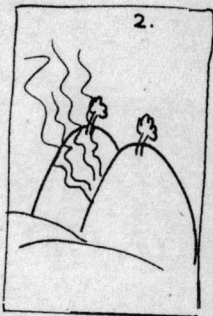

The Artist at Work

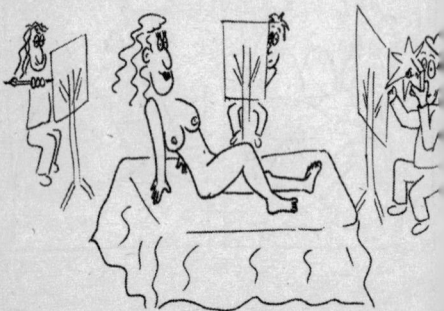

The Politician

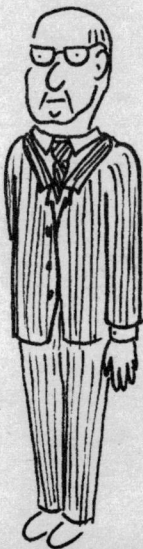

Traffic police

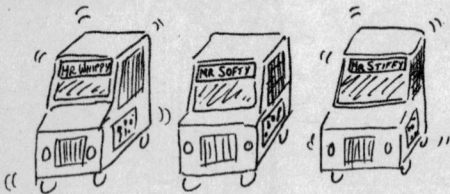

The Double Baton

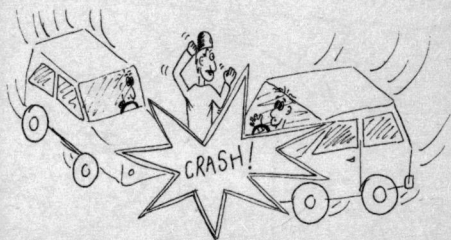

If you can't stand the heat . . .

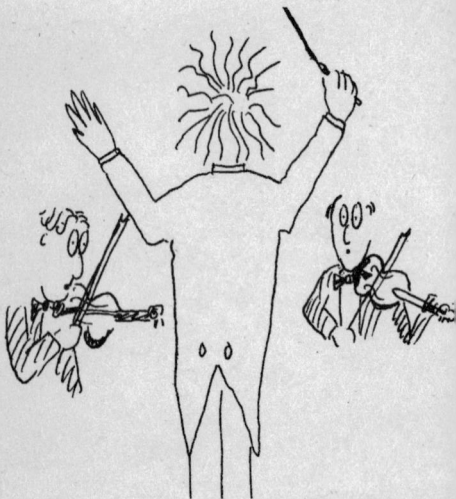

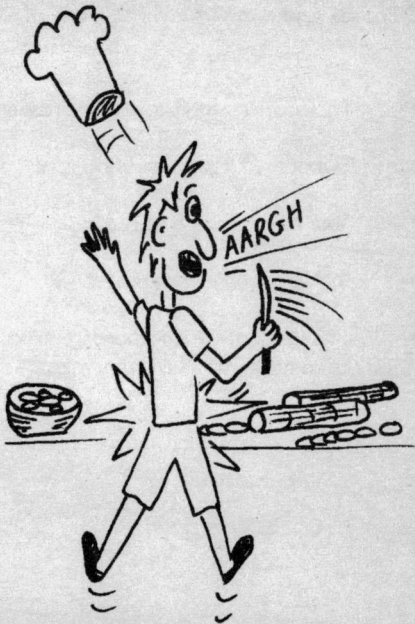

AARGH

Office sex toys

- Photocopier - see yourself from a new angle

- Swivel chairs - get yourself in a spin!

- Your boss's swivel chair (yuk)

- Vibrating mobile phone/pager

- Make your own rubber bondage suit out of office rubber bands and paperclips.

The Sport of Kings

Is sport better than sex? Or do real men prefer the sofa bed to the stadium? The answer is simple - sex is a sport. And, just like any other kind of sport, there will always be times when you just can't seem to field a team. But do not despair! Not only does the single man have more time for traditional sporting activities (ten pints down the pub in front of Sky), he can go in for the solo event and develop the natural sexual athlete inside him.

Training

Remember, you're not going out there to win any medals (although there is, of course, the Wankalympics, held every four years in Bent Baden, Germany, in which horny-handed athletes compete fiercely in a range of events: endurance, long jump, pole-vaulting and the climatic first across the line race). Take your training as seriously as you take your sport: stretches are vitally important if you want to avoid ligament damage and groin strains - a sharp pull or a sudden jerk when stiff can put you out of action for weeks.

My personal training regime is based on the late
developments in single male sports science. Initiall
the athlete lies in bed and exercises the abdomin
muscles by expressing the surplus gas produce
naturally by a high fat, low fibre diet (guys - th
vibrations also tone up that butt of yours!).

Next, attempt to raise yourself out of bed. If yo
can't manage this the first or second time, don't worr
Each attempt you make will tone and flex all the majc
muscle groups. Make sure, of course, that your hea
is the last part of you to leave the horizontal: this
best achieved by simply rolling out of bed, leadir
with your feet. Sticking your head to the pillow wit
saliva (if you're lucky) will make it even more of a
effort.

having achieved this warm-up routine, you feel
ready to launch straight into the main event, then go
for it - but don't expect to beat your personal best
first time off the blocks. Think of it more as a knock
about, a gallop in the park, just banging in a few shots
to get the feel of things. Then get to work on your
tackle, or other parts of your game that might need
some attention. It might be hard, but hard is what
you need to succeed, because the better you get,
the stiffer the opposition is going to be.

The Weight Lift

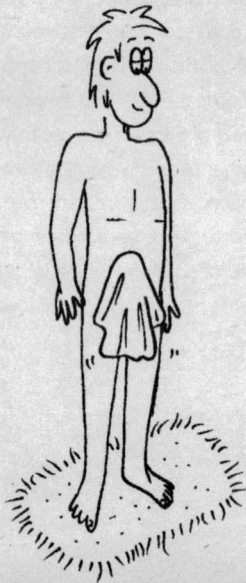

A jog to the bathroom is an excellent way of loosening rigid muscle groups, and may be supplemented by some squats. But do not overdo things. A sofa is a piece of sports equipment that is well worth investing in, and I find that a morning spent on the sofa or, for the most energetic, a reclining chair can make for an extremely effective work-out when combined with some 'personal fitness' videos. There are also some excellent magazines for the single fitness fan.

Testing your grip on the eigth hole

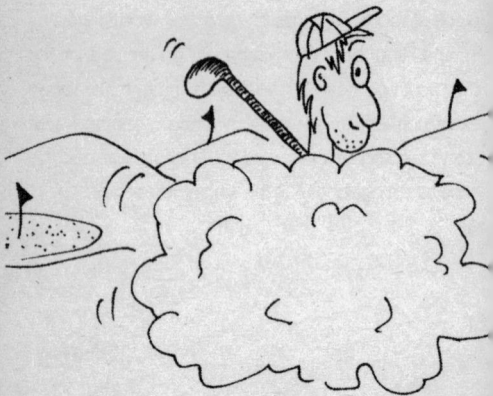

Potting the right balls

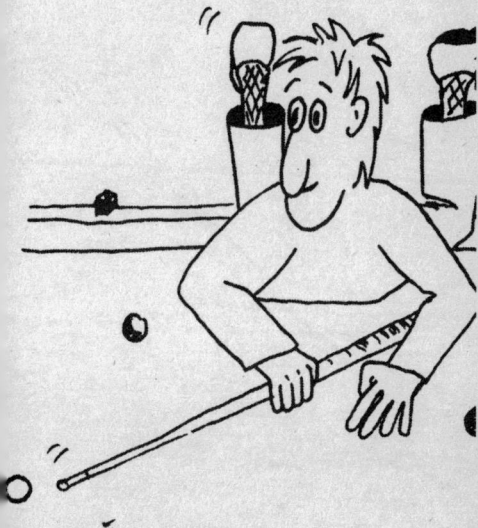

Groping for trouts in peculiar rivers

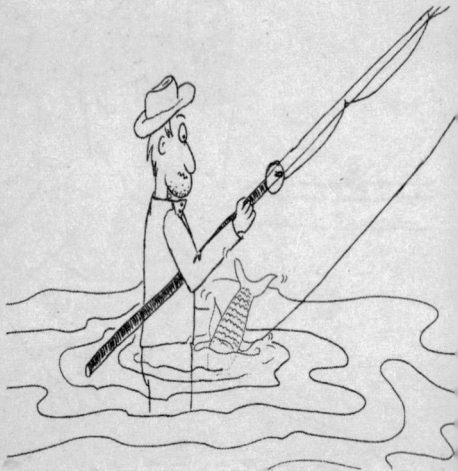

Water-sports

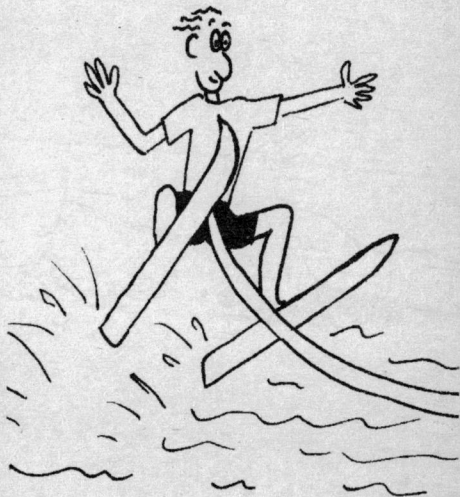

Riding the sea-sausage

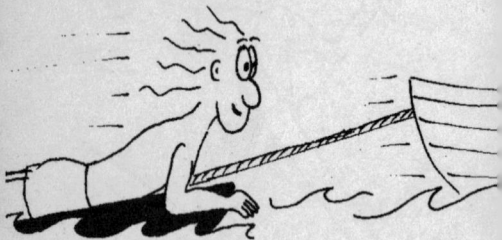

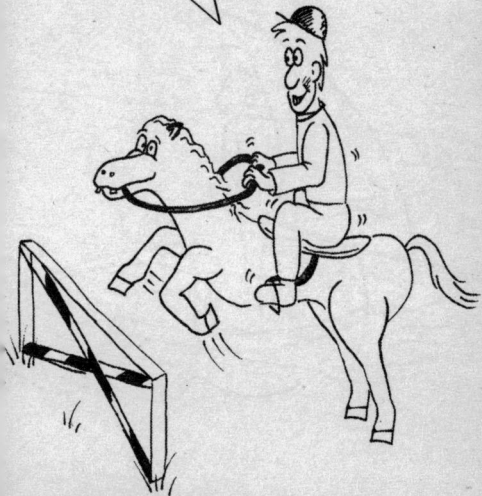

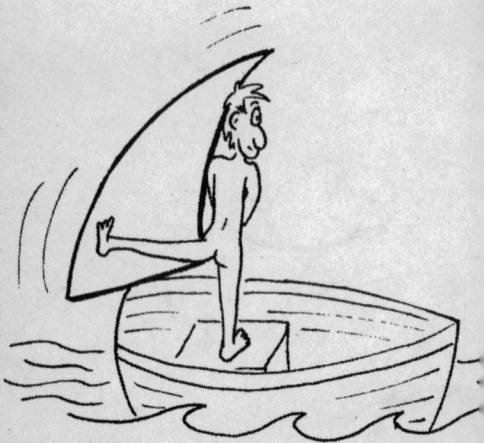

Pistol shooting

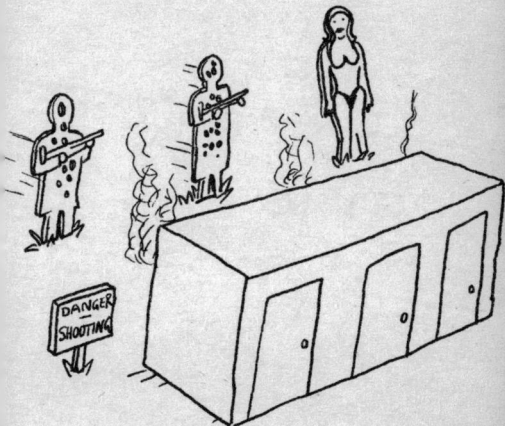

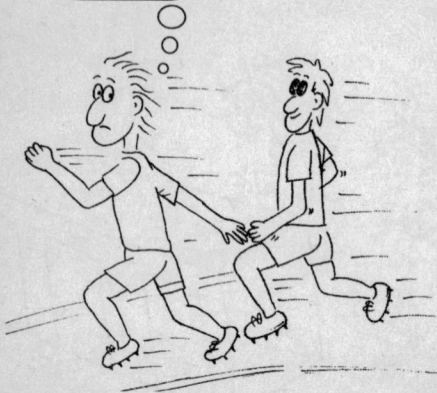

Time On
Your Hands

A man at rest is a happy man. It is our natural state. Think back for a moment to the times in life that you were happiest. Were you standing up? I don't think so. One thing that women have as yet largely failed to grasp is that there is no point working if you are not getting paid for it. And washing up, hoovering, cleaning the bath, cooking, and things like getting up to answer the phone count as work, unpaid labour. That is why there are things like pizza delivery, for instance.

Now, the man at rest is a man with time on his hands. Most of us who are on the path to single self-satisfaction are happy enough with a sofa, a quality magazine and a bog roll. But there is a whole world of leisure activity out there, and the truly committed leisure activist should not think that he must separate his single sex life from his leisure lifestyle.

For most people, an active leisure life involves the Great Outdoors - the parks, the fields and woods, the beach, the rivers and all that kind of stuff. Hardly the natural habitat for the traditional tosser. We have usually confined our activities to the hearth and home (though not literally the hearth, of course - though fire frotting is practised amongst the Swamis of Bangladore). But there is a wealth of opportunity out in the world of leisure activity for those who love themselves and, as I'm sure your mother told you, it's good to get it out in the fresh air.

This view may not be fully endorsed by law enforcement officers, and discretion is, as always, to be encouraged.

A range of concealment devices is available from all good men's outfitters. The most popular disguise for the out and about tosser is, of course, the taxi cab.

Reading the 'compass'

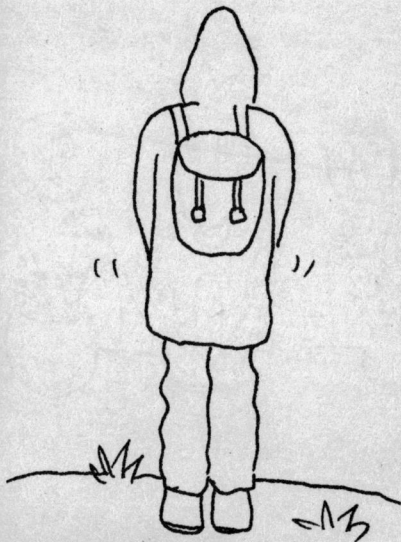

Flower arranging

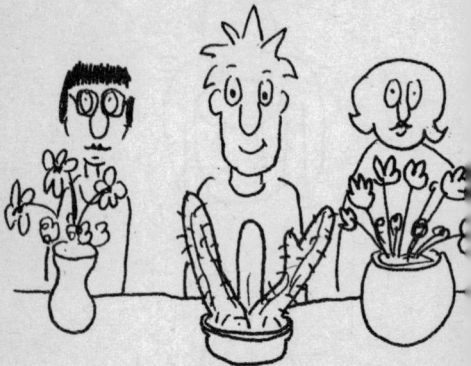

Ballroom dancing

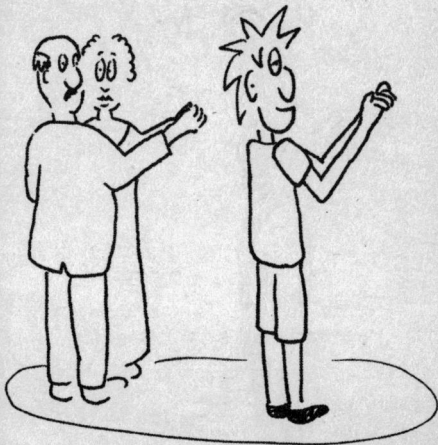

Back from a beach holiday

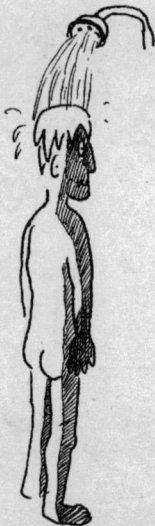

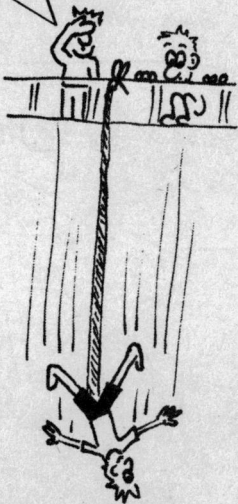

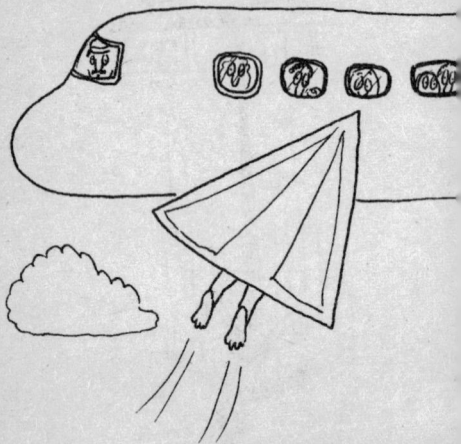

hang gliding

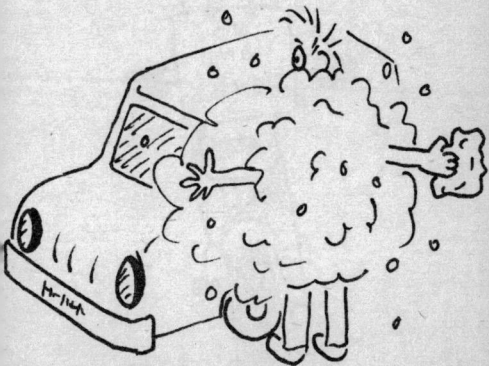

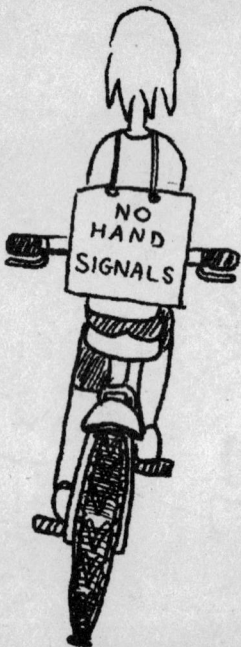

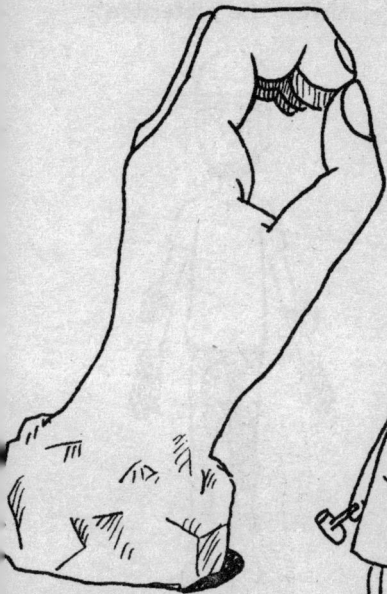
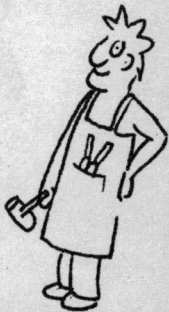

Always use protection

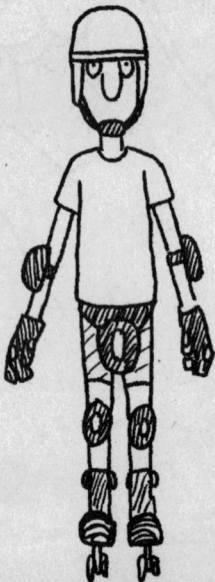

Bird watching

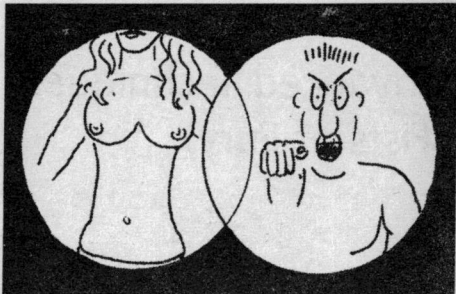

Advanced Techniques (Fists of Fury)

Every art has its great masters, and the art of self loving is no exception. The famous yanking yogies of California, for example, use an elaborate system of pulleys to stretch their manhoods by an inch a year - their older members have attained lengths of over six feet. The initiates of the Extreme Brotherhood devote themselves to month-long masturbatory marathons, while the Chilled Out Club sect freeze their members into foot-square ice blocks. Any decrease in tumescence leads to instant expulsion from all club social events.

All around the world, single men have set out to test the limits of their self-sex drive. Some have travelled to learn the secrets of the Far East (don't bother unless you can already lick behind your own ears), some have sought out remote or unusual locations where they really get in touch with themselves (such as Pete 'The Pole' Polakskii, who has been the subject of major police operations following his very public displays up national monuments in London, Paris, New York and Basildon). But most just go to Amsterdam for a long weekend.

How far you go depends on your tastes and life insurance policy. Non-solo sex has its share of 'adventurous' angles, and many single men have begun to grab the opportunities open to them with at least one hand.

Group sex

There is no real reason why stimulating yourself should be a solitary act, it all rather depends on the kind of company you keep. How well I remember those glorious days of my childhood at St Fistings Prep School, my chums and I gathered around a pothmug . . .

. . . but for those who relish the freedom from all inhibitions that total privacy brings, yet yearn for the frisson of group activity (or for those without broadminded chums), a large collection of mirrors gives a pleasingly well-populated effect. Several shop window dummies or life-size cardboard celebrities could also be used, but the sensitive self-pleasurer might find screen idols a bit intimidating.

Swinging/wife swapping

Try using your left hand (if right handed) or your right
hand (if left handed). Or your feet, to simulate you
best friend's sister-in-law.

Rubber fetishism

Easily satisfied by donning washing-up gloves - I find
store's own brands to be quite satisfactory.

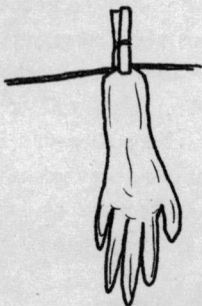

...le High Club

...tually a lot easier to achieve than if a partner is also ...volved. Whatever you do while in the air will almost ...rtainly never be as weird as what the person sitting ...xt to you will be up to.

...o the Khyber

...boxing glove (tightly gripped) and liberal usage of ...seline can be a remarkably lifelike experience. If ...u believe that it is better to receive than to give, ...en you can sort this one out for yourself.

...ndage

...od idea, but who's going to untie you?

Bestiality

Hand puppets of various attractive animals are ea[sily]
obtained from all good toy shops.

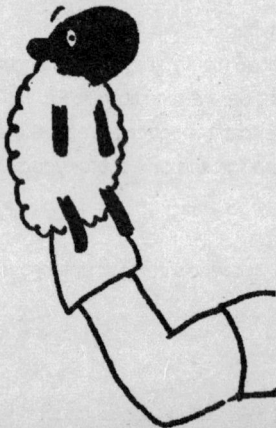

The best thing about masturbation, as this books has tried to show, is that it can be combined with all your favourite activities - watching TV, drinking beer, smoking, eating pizza - the list is, well, basically it's lots of things written one after another.

But if you try to combine your interests with non-solo sex, it leads to all kinds of problems and recriminations. Some women may be understanding about your need to watch the Grand Prix while servicing her needs, some may possibly enjoy your stopping to get a cold beer out of the fridge, or light a cigarette. But many others will surprise you with their loud and vehement objections.

Over-coming Obstacles

Excuses, Excuses

Man is a sexual animal - I know I am. But th
conjunction between our animalistic urges and th
conventions of modern society inevitably leads t
problems in every field of sexual behaviour. True, i
usually women who are to blame - they can be s
cruel about the smallest thing. But even those me
who are dedicated to loving only themselves ca
often find themselves in sticky situations.

So here are some of the most common obstacles
achieving self-satisfaction:

Failure to perform

Inevitably, this is linked to boyhood fears of discovery or the darker warnings about blindness, hairy palms or stunted growth. But think: you are now a grown man, successful, you can do what you like. Everyone thinks you're a wanker, anyway.

What about hairy palms, blindness or stunted growth?

All myths. And anyway there are plenty of depilatory creams, Braille readers and platform shoes to choose from.

Sexually transmitted disease

Everyone does it, so just be careful who you shake hands with. The truly paranoid find a pair of surgical gloves a great reassurance - with all the social rejection they bring with them.

Worrying fantasies

This is a surprisingly common phenomenon. Many men, for whatever reason, find they can only achieve release by imagining Jeremy Beadle astride a catering-size tin of ravioli, by picturing themselves amongst the penguins at London Zoo, or, more bizarrely, visualising their manhood trapped between Pamela Anderson's oiled and heaving breasts.

My advice, as a qualified TV psychologist, is to go along with these fantasies during the sexual act, and then feel extremely worried and guilty about them afterwards.

Frigidity

If the flesh is willing but the mind is not, then you are probably frigid.

I

Try romancing yourself with a bottle of wine and a good curry, tell yourself how special and marvellous you think you are, how adorable you look.

2

Laugh at your own jokes.

3

Let your mind relax until you are comfortable with yourself, then go for it before your mind realises that it's all just been a big trick for you to get what youb want out of it.

Works every time.

Obsession with talking about cars, sport and how great you are - this comes with the territory, I'm afraid.

Blistering and rawness

Eventually, your palm will become tough and calloused and up to the fastest action you can throw at it. You really want to avoid the same happening to your John Thomas, however. As with heavy machinery, a spot of lubrication keeps everything working smoothly. I recommend chip fat.

Inability to stop masturbating

This isn't a problem; this is normal male behaviour.

Buying pornography

Study the following diagram for buying jazz mags.

1. Select newspaper

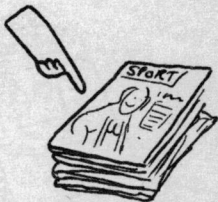

2. Quick as a flash, grab mag off shelf and put inside newspaper

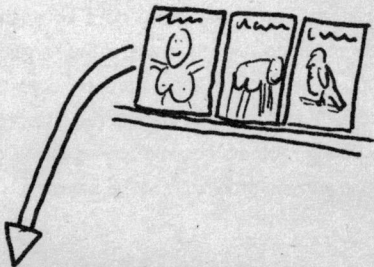

3. Arrange things so that just the top of the mag is sticking out, and take it up to the till.

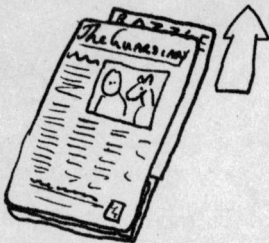

It used to work, but these days you can't get shopkeepers to keep their side of the bargain: they either accuse you of shop lifting or expose your purchase - to the gasps and muttered disapproval of the young mothers and old crones in the queue behind you - in order to read the bar code.

Getting a girlfriend - Sometimes this is simply unavoidable. You go out single, get drunk, then wake up to a short engagement for a spring wedding.

You can try to continue just pleasing yourself, but it is more than likely that this will lead to physical and emotional suffering - almost all by you. Or you could try explaining your need to express yourself: but this is also almost certainly doomed to failure. For some unknown reason, women find something distasteful about their partners sneaking away for a quick one off the wrist, let alone a long and satisfying session with your magazine lovelies. So you will have to be discrete. This probably means the bathroom, but don't take too long. She'll know.

Other Humour Books from Summersdale

Available from all good bookshops.

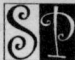

How To Chat-up Women (Pocket edition)	£3.99
How To Chat-up Men (Pocket edition)	£3.99
Enormous Boobs *The Greatest Mistakes In The History of the World*	£4.99
101 Uses for a Losing Lottery Ticket	£3.99
Men! Can't Live with them, Can't live *with* them	£3.99
www.wit@wisdom	£4.99
Drinking Games	£3.99
Girl Power	£3.99
Ultimate Chat-up Lines	£3.99
101 Reasons Not To Do Anything *A Collection of Cynical & Defeatist Quotations*	£3.99
A Little Bathroom Book	£3.99
101 Reasons why it's Great to be a Woman	£3.99